SUGAR DETOX

THE 21 DAY METHOD

Antoine L. Miller

Contents

Chapter One

Introduction

Holistic nutrition is my specialty, and I'm a board-certified nutritionist. I've also had issues with sugar and carb cravings, just like you. I, too, had a hard time breaking through to sugar-freedom since sugar is so potent. But I've figured out how to fix this enormous problem, and it makes me happier than I've ever been!

In response to the growing number of people on the lookout for a more healthful way of living, I created The 21-Day Sugar Detox programme. At some point in my career, I've worked with a huge number of individuals and groups that have been plagued by sugar and carbohydrate cravings. In fact, I started my practise with the goal of helping people like you by focusing on blood sugar regulation.

Whether you're a busy mom or a high-level athlete looking to curb your sugar cravings, the 21-Day Sugar Detox is for you. For anyone who wants to feel better, have more energy and a better night's sleep, and stop riding the blood sugar roller coaster all day long (you know, the trip you're on when your meals and snacks are high in carbs and low in vitamins and minerals), this book is for you.

In a world where contradicting diet advice comes at us from every angle—from television doctors, magazines, the evening news, and even your hairdresser!—it's no wonder you haven't found out how to regulate your urges yet. Sugar is bad for you, and you've probably already read a lot of books about that. But those books don't show you how to stop eating it. You get precisely that with the 21-Day Sugar Detox: a concise, practical approach for breaking free from the chains of sugar and carbs.

About the Sugar Detox for 21 Days

21DSD is an all-natural, whole-foods-based programme that aims to help you rethink your eating habits, your taste buds, and your entire connection with the food you eat every day. You won't be able to look at the meals you previously ate the same way after three weeks of following The 21DSD "Yes" list. As you become more conscious of the effects particular foods have on your body and mind, your habits will begin to shift. Sweets can leave you feeling drowsy, moody, and out of whack.

Many people, for good reason, lose their enthusiasm within the first few days of a nutritional reset or detox programme.

To get the results you want, most diets call for you to restrict your caloric intake, take pills, or drink shakes and juices all day long. The 21-Day Sugar Detox is not about that at all. It's not what your body needs when you're seeking for a fresh start—clean, nutritious, whole foods that are rich in nutrients are what it requires. The body's natural detoxification system works best when nutrients such as protein, fat, and vitamins and minerals are present in sufficient quantities in each meal. You see, your body was designed to be self-cleaning. However, this is nothing more than simple biology at work. However, you must feed your body real food in order to complete the detox process. Period.

Why do you need to cut out sugar from your diet?

Sugar is a sly thief. When consumed in excess, excessive consumption can lead to numerous health problems, both short-term and long-term. Symptoms of sugar addiction are well-known to most of us, including excessive energy surges and dips, as well as that nagging feeling that you're not fulfilled until you have a sweet fix. Sugar's negative consequences, however, extend far further. Toxic effects of nutrition-poor carbohydrate overconsumption include the following less-obvious symptoms: sugar cravings, blood sugar swings, and vitamin shortages.

IMMEDIATE RESULTS

Mood changes

Acne, rashes

As a result of premenstrual syndrome (PMS), menstrual cramps

Anxiety-inducing dreams

- Fatigue
- Weakness or exhaustion of the muscles
- Cold and flu susceptibility

Other food-related compulsions are also possible.

CONSIDERATIONS FOR THE FUTURE

- Anemia
- Anxiety and depression

Cystic acne, eczema, and psoriasis

PCOS, infertility

- Insomnia

Adrenal exhaustion or malfunction may be to blame.

Disabilities of the visual system

Disorders of the nervous system

- Type 2 diabetes, insulin resistance, and obesity

- Alzheimer's
- Addiction to drugs

Whatever we think, sugar is encroaching on our daily life. Because of our addiction to sugary and carbohydrate-rich foods, we've almost become captives to the blood sugar roller coaster. To be clear, this does not mean that all carbs are harmful. Vegetables and fruits, which are high in carbohydrate, are wonderful things, but we all know that they aren't the kinds of foods that drive us to go into a sugar coma and race to the next candy bowl. "Good carbs," as I refer to them, are the reason. In addition to providing your body with the energy it requires, carbohydrates also provide your body with essential nutrients such as vitamins and minerals. In order to get a better grasp on the subject of good carbs vs. bad carbs, I suggest going back and rereading the first section of The 21-Day Sugar Detox guidebook.

This cookbook's unique selling point

My first book in this series, The 21-Day Sugar Detox, serves as a companion and a supplement to this cuisine. After many years of operating the programme without printed materials for participants, I decided it was time to make this information available in a much larger, better method. The 21-Day Sugar Detox is a compilation of my finest sugar-busting tips.

the following is included in the guidebook:

• the science behind why we crave sugar and what it does to our bodies

how to get ready

detailed information about what to expect on a daily basis

Tips & strategies for repurposing leftovers and eating out

• how to get aid and support as you go

• over 90 delicious and quick recipes

Yes, there are numerous recipes included in the guidebook as a whole. In the previous several years, I've learnt that preparation and inspiring meals are the keys to your success on The 21DSD!

Over a hundred additional healthy and delectable sugar-free recipes, as well as gluten-free, grain-free, dairy-free, and Paleo-friendly options, are included in this volume. You'll want to eat a lot more food while on the 21-Day Sugar Detox, but finding 21DSD-friendly recipes for those meals can be difficult. For individuals with egg allergies or sensitivities, there are more egg-free breakfast options in this book, as well as more delectable main courses, sides, snacks, and not-so-sweet desserts to tantalise your taste buds. Additionally, I've created more sugar-detox-friendly versions of your favourite dressings and sauces, along with a variety of spice blends to keep your plate bursting with flavour (without the added sugars and chemical preservatives found in most commercial varieties) regardless of whether you follow a specific recipe or not. This is your secret weapon and express train to Flavor Town!

During The 21-Day Sugar Detox, you will notice a dramatic shift in your palate's response to food. Foods that didn't appear very sweet the first several days can suddenly feel incredibly sweet. Even if you made a not-sweet dish on Day 1, it will taste significantly better on Day 7. In this book, I show you how to take advantage of this change in your taste senses. While you won't be using concentrated sweeteners like honey or maple syrup while on The 21DSD, many of these recipes use items like caramelised onions and cooked-down green apples in sauces and dishes that you would normally sweeten with honey or maple syrup. BBQ sauce, honey-free mustard, and sweetener-free ketchup are all on the menu. All those extra sweeteners you've given up will not be missed for a second.

Concerning the menus

Three 21-day meal plans based on the book's recipes are included in the 21-Day Sugar Detox handbook. This cookbook uses only recipes from this book in the same way. With the help of these meal plans, you'll be able to round up your 21DSD with more options, resources, and ideas. Whether you're embarking on a 21-Day Sugar Detox for the first time or returning for a second time, I've got you covered.

Now, you may be wondering why someone would desire or need to do The 21DSD a second or third time. You may assume that the goal is to eliminate your cravings forever and ever. That's exactly what happens to a lot of folks! They can be life-changing in just three weeks. Some people return to The 21DSD to provide a hand to a friend or loved one who is going through a detox. Attempting a nutritional reset more than once a year (and maybe at an even higher level) presents a new set of obstacles and consequences for some people, especially those who begin the programme at Level 1.

In the event that your sugar intake has veered off course, I encourage you to revisit The 21DSD. However, even though the 21DSD programme is designed to limit your sugar cravings in just three weeks, you may discover that following the holidays, you need a post-holiday 21DSD to get yourself back on track.

About those recipes...

In this book, the recipes are broken down into the following categories:

• Main Dishes

Side dishes, soups, and salads

- Snacks
- Snacks That Aren't Sweet

Food Additives & Condiments

- Basics of Cooking

A wide range of recipes for a wide range of tastes and preferences can be found in each department. Even if you don't make every meal in this book, you'll still have a great time cooking your way through it and be successful in your detox.

Egg-free breakfasts appear first in the Main Dishes section, followed by those that include eggs. The following is a list of chicken, red meat, pork, and seafood/meat-free choices. In many cases, the main dishes and accompanying side dishes were designed in tandem, although you are free to mix and match them as you choose.

A wide selection of options are available in the next section of the menu, including soups, salads, and side dishes. Adapt the recipes in this book to suit your own tastes and preferences, or come up with your own unique concoctions from the ones provided.

This year, I've put together a new batch of savoury recipes that can be made ahead of time and stored in the fridge or freezer for those times when hunger strikes.

The 21-Day Sugar Detox programme is known for its not-so-sweet goodies. It may be difficult to give up some of your favourite foods for three weeks, but once you try these new versions, you'll be glad you did. These recipes are packed with foods that nourish your body while soothing your mind, so don't worry if they don't taste as good on Day 1 as they will in the following days (since, as I indicated before, your tastes will change—and I am banking on that for you!).

The Kitchen Basics portion of the book contains recipes that you can use as a foundation for the rest of the book's meals. Forget the pre-packaged and canned versions of these dishes; they'll have you wondering why you ever bought them in the first place.

Putting the instructions to good use

In this book and the handbook, each recipe is suitable for all three levels of the programme and comprises multiple components. You'll find all the anticipated details, such as how long the dish takes to prepare, the ingredients used, the method of preparation, and the number of servings it makes. In addition, you'll get useful advice on ingredients, cooking methods, and even the equipment you'll need to get started. There are some ingredients in the recipes I've identified because I know how important it is for many of you to stay away from those that are known to cause allergies or irritation. When it comes to some ingredients, I've even provided you advice on how to leave them out if you're trying to avoid certain foods. Check out the recommendations in the recipe boxes, or look here for a comprehensive list of ingredient replacements to use when avoiding common allergens.

Cooking from a guidebook means you'll certainly come across some new ingredients, so be prepared! (or my first book, Practical Paleo). Here is a list of specific components that you may learn more about, including what they are, why you should include them in your diet, and how much you should eat while on the programme. To help you get started on your new diet, we've put together a list of recommended products and brands that you can use during and after your detox.

Components and how to use them in a recipe

Extraordinary substances

a list of some of the more common ingredients in this book's plot

Products made from almonds

What Is It?

Peanut or cashew butter can be swapped out for this creamy almond butter.

Is there a good reason to do this?

Nuts and cashews are not included in the 21DSD diet.

Is it a lot?

While on The 21DSD, I advise you to use almond and other nut butters sparingly (walnut, pecan, hazelnut). If you prepare too many almond butter-based products or don't serve yourself in moderation, you may find yourself overindulging and developing bad habits. Serving sizes are included in all of the recipes in this book that use almond butter.

CORN STARCH

What Is It?

A substitute for wheat or other grain flours that behaves nearly identically in baking.

What's the point of doing it this way anyway?

There are no grain flours in the 21DSD scheme.

How much is this going to cost?

While on The 21DSD, I advise you to use almond and other nut flours sparingly. If you bake too many almond flour-based products, you may find yourself overindulging and developing bad habits. There is no specific amount of almond flour that you may safely consume. All of the almond flour treat recipes in this book include information on serving sizes.

Eating an almond meal is a good idea.

What Is It?

Texture and crunch can be added to recipes by substituting it for wheat flour or other grain meal.

What's the point of doing it this way anyway?

There are no grain flours or meals included in the 21DSD programme.

How much is this going to cost?

While on The 21DSD, I recommend that you limit your consumption of almond and other nut meals.

APPLE CIDER VINEGAR.

What Is It?

The fermentation of apples yields an apple vinegar. Make sauces and dressings using it.

What's the point of doing it this way anyway?

Gluten-free and a natural digestion aid, it is an excellent choice.

How much is this going to cost?

On The 21DSD, you can use as much apple cider vinegar as you like.

BUTTER & GHEE CLARIFIED

What Is It?

When the solids in whole butter are removed and cooked, the result is a pure form of butterfat. It's clarified butter taken one step farther in the process (see here for details).

What's the point of doing it this way anyway?

In comparison to butter, it is more heat-resistant.

How much is this going to cost?

All of your clarified butter and ghee can be used throughout the 21DSD.

AMINOS FROM COCONUT

What Is It?

A substance made from fermented coconut sap. Like soy sauce, it can be used in any recipe calling for soy sauce.

What's the point of doing it this way anyway?

The 21DSD does not include soy, and this is a substitute for soy sauce. For those who are sensitive to gluten, this is a better option than soy sauce.

How much is this going to cost?

Coconut aminos can be used quite generously.

COCONUT BUTTER.

What Is It?

Finely ground coconut meat is used to create this nut butter-like spread.

What's the point of doing it this way anyway?

In the event that you are allergic to nuts, coconut butter can be used as an alternative to nut butter in many recipes.

How much is this going to cost?

Any amount of coconut butter you want to consume each day is fine; more than two tablespoons is probably too much.

FLOUR FROM COCONUT

What Is It?

Coconut flour is a high-fiber flour created by grinding coconut meat into a fine powder.

What's the point of doing it this way anyway?

The 21DSD excludes grain flours. Coconut flour is an excellent substitute for nut flours if you are allergic to nuts or simply don't want to bake with them.

What's the total cost?

Coconut flour should only be used sparingly, in my opinion. Understand that it can't be used in recipes that call for other flours in the same way as regular flour. In order to get a moist result with coconut flour, you'll typically need to use more eggs than you would with other flours.

Chapter Two

Good foods for you

MILK OF CONGO

What Is It?

Non-dairy milk that may either be prepared at home or purchased in cans (see here for a recipe). Because of the huge quantity of additives in the cartons, I do not suggest this product.

What's the point of doing it this way anyway?

For those who are lactose or casein intolerant, vegan, or on the third level of the 21DSD, coconut milk is an option. It is excellent in Asian dishes since it enhances the flavour and fat content.

How much is this going to cost?

Although coconut milk is permitted on The 21DSD, I don't recommend consuming more than 8 ounces each day.

OIL FROM COCOA BEAN

What Is It?

Saturated fat that may be utilised in both sweet and savoury foods is called coconut oil.

What's the point of doing it this way anyway?

As a result, it is suitable for cooking at high temperatures and for making sweets and other desserts.

How much is this going to cost?

While on The 21DSD, there is no restriction to the amount of coconut oil you can consume.

SESEA OIL COLD-PRESSED

What Is It?

Whole sesame seeds are pressed into oil using a cold-pressing technique.

What's the point of doing it this way anyway?

Finishing up Asian meals with it brings out their full flavour even more fully than they would have without it.

How much is this going to cost?

While on The 21DSD, there is no restriction to the amount of sesame oil you can consume.

Olive oil that is extra-virgin

What Is It?

This is the initial pressing oil from olives.

What's the point of doing it this way anyway?

Vitamin E and polyphenols are among the many nutrients it contains.

How much is this going to cost?

The 21DSD has no limit on the amount of olive oil you can consume.

FISH SAUCE

What Is It?

Traditional Asian cuisine relies heavily on the use of a salt-fermented fish sauce.

What's the point of doing it this way anyway?

It enhances the flavour of Asian cuisine and serves as a foundation for the umami flavour.

How much is this going to cost?

While on The 21DSD, there is no restriction to the amount of fish sauce you can consume.

GELATIN

What Is It?

A powdered collagen derivative from animal bones, such as pig or cow, typically.

What's the point of doing it this way anyway?

To put it simply, it holds everything together, but it's more important to note that it's an excellent source of glycine, collagen, and protein.

How much is this going to cost?

While on The 21DSD, there is no limit to the amount of gelatin you can consume.

TAHINI SAME

What Is It?

As a substitute for peanut or other nut/seed butters, sesame paste is commonly used in savoury foods like soups and stews.

What's the point of doing it this way anyway?

Seed-based snacks may be a good option for those who are allergic to nuts.

How much is this going to cost?

While on The 21DSD, I advise you to exercise caution when it comes to using seed butters. There isn't a predetermined limit.

SUNBUTTER

What Is It?

Peanut, cashew, and other nut butter substitutes can be created from pulverised sunflower seeds.

What's the point of doing it this way anyway?

Seed-based snacks may be a good option for those who are allergic to nuts.

How much is this going to cost?

While on The 21DSD, I advise you to exercise caution when it comes to using seed butters. If you prepare too many sunbutter-based products or don't control portion sizes, you may end up overindulging and developing bad habits. Sunbutter-based treats in this book all include serving sizes.

Is it a food that makes you say "Yes"?

Following the instructions and Yes/No Foods Lists provided in the following pages, you may come across foods not included in the programme or be unsure whether a specific food is allowed or not. Following these guidelines will help you decide whether or not a food is appropriate for your current level of health and wellness.

- Sweeteners of any kind are not permitted. If you want a taste of sweetness, you'll have to eat the fruits featured in your "Yes/No Foods" list in moderation. If a packaged food item's ingredients list has an additional sweetener, you can't eat it. Full-fat dairy products on Levels 1 and 2 contain natural sugars, which are fine to consume. In order to eat bacon that contains sugar, the total carbs per serving must be less than 1 gramme.

• It's not allowed if it's sweet and isn't on your level's list of Yes or Limit meals. Herbal teas that have a naturally sweet flavour are permitted. Don't include anything that tastes sweet but you're not sure about.

It is not permitted to use grain flours. Foods manufactured with whole-grain or refined-grain flours will not be consumed (wheat, spelt, and quinoa flours, for example). Some limited starches and flours from nuts and seeds are permitted (like tapioca or arrowroot flour when used as a thickening agent in sauces).

1. GET A GOOD NIGHT'S SLEEP. You're setting yourself up for a full day of cravings if you don't get enough sleep.

Drinking water is a good way to stay hydrated. If you think you're hungry, it's probably just your body telling you that you're dehydrated.

Be prepared. When you're prepared with the correct foods, you're more likely to be able to resist cravings and yet have nutritious food on hand should one occur.

ADD A FRIEND TO YOUR TEAM. You might think of a friend, a coworker, a member of your family, or someone else. Having the support of a person you spend a lot of time with on a daily basis can go a long way toward completing this goal.

HERBAL TEA IS A DELICIOUS DRINK. If you're looking for a caffeine-free beverage, herbal tea is your best bet. You won't feel deprived if you have a yearning because it's usually a special occasion.

Fat, then protein, then vegetables. How to construct a plate, whether it's for dinner or dessert.

7. MAKE SNACKS OUT OF YOUR MEALS. Make a little extra when you're cooking and keep any leftovers in a container in case you need them as a snack. It doesn't have to be "snack food" to be a snack.

Take a stroll. If you're tempted by something delicious, try something else to take your mind off of things.

CAFFEINE MUST BE REDUCED. Sugar cravings are exacerbated by caffeine. Reduce your coffee intake for the first week if you're having trouble sleeping.

Relax! Sugar cravings will only be exacerbated if you're worried about the detox!

Chapter Three

Planning your meal schedule

You can follow this meal plan to the letter, tweak it to fit your preferences, or simply follow the Yes/No Foods List here and these general remarks while doing the 21-Day Sugar Detox at Level 1.

On some days, you can omit the following foods from your meals or snacks if you like. The meal plan's optional components are highlighted in bold italics.

Whole grain and legumes

Cooked up to half a cup a day

This programme is restricted to the use of gluten-free grains.

- amaranth
- arrowroot
- beans include black, fava, navy, pinto, red

- buckwheat

Beans in the garbanzo variety (chickpeas)

- lentils
- millet
- quinoa
- a grain of rice (white, brown, wild)
- sorghum
- tapioca

Whole-grain items (such brown rice pasta and whole-grain cereals) are excluded from this list.

This meal plan incorporates grains and beans to meet your daily 1/2 cup recommendation depending on the types of cuisine and flavour combinations.

If you're not strictly following the meal plan, you'll have to figure out where to put your 1/2 cup serving. The recipes in this book are suitable for cooks of all skill levels because they don't call for the use of grains or legumes.

When you eat your share, you are free to make adjustments. At example, if you plan to eat rice for lunch but choose to have additional carbs for dinner, you can do so. Overall, I've found that eating carbs later in the day helps me sleep better and keeps my blood sugar levels more consistent throughout the day.

DAIRY WITH A LOT OF FAT no section of the body is restricted

Products with less than 2% fat content in milk are prohibited.

It can be made from a wide variety of foods such as:

half-and-half; • whole milk; • heavy cream;

yoghurt or kefir that is simple and full-fat

salt and pepper to taste

It's up to you whether or not you want to eat full-fat dairy on a regular basis. Here are some ideas for where to put it in your strategy. Whenever feasible, purchase local, grass-fed, and non-homogenized products. If you can't locate grass-fed dairy, organic is the best option.

Yoga alone does not require these modifications, but you may need them if you engage in high-intensity physical activity or exercise regularly (for example, interval training, CrossFit-style workouts, endurance athletics, or cardio/aerobic activity at moderate to high intensity for more than 20 minutes at a time).

have recently given birth to a child

Your share of whole grains and legumes will increase as a result of the Energy Modifications. Those who do not meet the dietary modifications outlined above will need to include starchy carbohydrate vegetables such as potatoes and corn in their meal plan.

Whole grain and legumes

up to 1 cup of cooked oat bran each day

According to your Yes/No Foods List, you've set a maximum number of calories per day that you're willing to eat.

VEGETABLES HIGH IN STARCH-INDUCED CARBOHYDRATE

Depending on how active you are and how much energy you need, the amount of these meals you should eat can be found here.

One meal a day, especially after exercise, should include 30–50 grammes of carbohydrates. So, for example, you may use half to a cup of mashed sweet potato. All Level 1 detoxers are required to eat one piece of fruit per day in order to meet this carbohydrate goal.

Train hard (at high intensity or more than once daily) and you may need to make this adjustment for each activity, which means up to 30-50 grammes of dense carbs in many meals and snacks.

Adjust the time of day you eat your additional carbs. If sweet potato is on the menu for lunch, but you choose to eat your additional carbs after dinner, that is perfectly OK as well. Late in the day or after a workout is generally the best time to refuel your body with carbohydrates. Tracking your personal energy levels is the greatest approach to figure out when to eat more carbs in your meal plan.

Recommendation for Carbohydrate Consumption per Day

75–150 grammes of activity

100–200 grammes of highly active protein

100+ grammes if you're pregnant or nursing.

Estimates are based on the information available at the time. Adjust your carbohydrate intake if you find yourself unable to maintain your activity level.

Consider adding these carbohydrate sources if you are pregnant or nursing. Don't limit them in the hope of improving outcomes. It is not required to restrict these items any farther in order to achieve the program's goal of a healthy body and healthy baby. In the event that your milk production is less than usual, or you're feeling more tired than usual, try increasing your consumption of carbohydrate-dense foods.

additional information for vegetarians and vegans who do not consume meat, eggs, or dairy products

THIS CHANGE MAY BE PERFECT FOR YOU, IF

• Adopt a pescetarian eating pattern.

With the Pescetarian Modifications, you'll eat more whole grains and legumes in your diet. Those who do not meet the dietary modifications outlined above will need to include starchy carbohydrate vegetables such as potatoes and corn in their meal plan.

Whole grain and legumes

You can eat up to 1 cup of cooked vegetables each day.

According to your Yes/No Foods List, you've set a maximum number of calories per day that you're willing to eat. If you're getting enough protein and carbs from other sources, you don't need to eat the recommended grains or legumes every day.

VEGETABLES HIGH IN STARCH-INDUCED CARBOHYDRATE

For a complete list of these foods, click here.

DAIRY WITH A LOT OF FAT no section of the body is restricted

If you want to up the protein and fat content of your meals, consider including some high-quality dairy products. Whenever feasible, purchase local, grass-fed, and non-homogenized products. If you can't locate grass-fed dairy, organic is the best option.

ADDITIONAL FATS

increase the amount of fat in your meals and snacks

As an illustration:

use an entire avocado instead of a half in a dinner

• substitute 1/4 cup nuts and/or dressing for 2 tablespoons in a salad

dairy products can be a helpful source of fat and protein if you are able to tolerate them without experiencing symptoms like gas, bloating, digestive irritation or breakouts.

SEAFOOD

At the very least, include seafood as a protein source in two of your daily meals.

You may opt to follow this meal plan to the letter, modify it to fit your personal preferences, or simply follow the Yes/No Foods List here and these general remarks while doing the 21-Day Sugar Detox at Level 2.

On some days, you can omit the following foods from your meals or snacks if you like. The meal plan's optional components are highlighted in bold italics.

DAIRY WITH A LOT OF FAT

no section of the body is restricted

Dairy products that are low in fat or nonfat are not permitted.

It can be made from a wide variety of foods such as:

half-and-half; • whole milk; • heavy cream;

yoghurt or kefir that is simple and full-fat

salt and pepper to taste

It's up to you whether or not you want to eat full-fat dairy on a regular basis. There are a few places where you can incorporate it into the following approach. Whenever feasible, purchase local, grass-fed, and non-homogenized products. If you can't locate grass-fed dairy, organic is the best option.

For those who require extra carbohydrates, here are some more remarks

If you have a physically demanding profession or have an active lifestyle, these modifications may be ideal for you.

For example, interval training, CrossFit-style workouts, endurance athletics or cardio/aerobic activities at moderate to high intensity for more than 20 minutes at a time (yoga alone doesn't normally require these changes; these adaptations are not necessary for yoga).

have recently given birth to a child

You'll need to include starchy carbohydrate veggies to your meal plan as part of the Energy Modifications if you don't meet the modification requirements.

VEGETABLES HIGH IN STARCH-INDUCED CARBOHYDRATE

Depending on how active you are and how much energy you need, the amount of these meals you should eat can be found here.

One meal a day, especially after exercise, should include 30–50 grammes of carbohydrates. Sweet potato or plantain, for example, can be mashed into a half- to one-cup portion. Carbohydrate intake must be met by consuming a single piece of fruit per day for all Level 2 detoxers.

This alteration may be necessary if you train really hard (at high intensity or more than once a day), therefore more than one meal or snack may contain up to this amount of dense carbohydrates.

Adjust the time of day you eat your additional carbs. If sweet potato is on the menu for lunch, but you choose to eat your additional carbs after dinner, that is perfectly OK as well. Late in the day or after a workout is generally the best time to refuel your body with carbohydrates. Tracking your personal energy levels is the greatest approach to figure out when to eat more carbs in your meal plan.

Recommendation for Carbohydrate Consumption per Day

75–150 grammes of activity

100–200 grammes of highly active protein

100+ grammes if you're pregnant or nursing.

Estimates are based on the information available at the time. Adjust your carbohydrate intake if you find yourself unable to maintain your activity level.

Consider adding these carbohydrate sources if you are pregnant or nursing. Don't limit them in the hope of improving outcomes. It is not required to restrict these items any farther in order to achieve the program's goal of a healthy body and healthy baby. In the event that your milk production is less than usual, or you're feeling more tired than usual, try increasing your consumption of carbohydrate-dense foods.

additional information for vegetarians and vegans who do not consume meat, eggs, or dairy products

THIS CHANGE MAY BE PERFECT FOR YOU

• Adopt a pescetarian eating pattern.

You'll get more whole grains and legumes if you follow the Pescetarian diet. For those who don't meet the modification requirements above, you'll need to include starchy carbohydrate veggies in your diet plan.

VEGETABLES HIGH IN STARCH-INDUCED CARBOHYDRATE

up to two cups may be consumed each day; For a complete list of these foods, click here.

DAIRY WITH A LOT OF FAT

no section of the body is restricted

If you want to up the protein and fat content of your meals, consider including some high-quality dairy products. Whenever feasible, purchase local, grass-fed, and non-homogenized products. If you can't locate grass-fed dairy, organic is the best option.

ADDITIONAL FATS

increase the amount of fat in your meals and snacks

As an illustration:

use an entire avocado instead of a half in a dinner

• substitute 1/4 cup nuts and/or dressing for 2 tablespoons in a salad

dairy products can be a helpful source of fat and protein if you are able to tolerate them without experiencing symptoms like gas, bloating, digestive irritation or breakouts.

SEAFOOD

at least one and preferably two meals a day should contain seafood as the primary protein source

INTERACTIVE MEAL PLANNING

You can follow this meal plan to the letter, tweak it to suit your preferences, or simply follow the Yes/No Foods List here and these general remarks while doing the 21-Day Sugar Detox at Level 3.

This level has the fewest options for food. Because some people like the “hardest” or “strictest” programme, it’s not a good idea to attempt Level 3. Your answers to the quiz here indicated that this is the best course of action for you, thus you should have ended up here.

What distinguishes Level 3 from the other two levels?

All cereals and dairy products are banned from Level 3. The Paleo diet is often used to describe this kind of eating plan. My book Practical Paleo is a good introduction to this way of eating. The 21DSD differs from a regular Paleo diet in that it removes extra natural sugars and sweet-tasting foods in an effort to improve your eating patterns.

Yoga alone does not require these modifications, but you may need them if you engage in high-intensity physical activity or exercise regularly (for example, interval training, CrossFit-style workouts, endurance athletics, or cardio/aerobic activity at moderate to high intensity for more than 20 minutes at a time).

have recently given birth to a child

You’ll need to include starchy carbohydrate veggies to your meal plan as part of the Energy Modifications if you don’t meet the modification requirements.

VEGETABLES HIGH IN STARCH-INDUCED CARBOHYDRATE

Depending on how active you are and how much energy you need, the amount of these meals you should eat can be found here.

One meal a day, especially after exercise, should include 30–50 grammes of carbohydrates. Sweet potato or plantain, for example, can be mashed into a half- to one-cup portion. All Level 3 detoxers are required to consume one piece of fruit per day in order to meet their daily carbohydrate goal.

To get the most out of your training, you may need to increase your carbohydrate intake by up to 30–50 grammes per meal or snack if you work out frequently or at a high intensity.

Adjust the time of day you eat your additional carbs. If sweet potato is on the menu for lunch, but you choose to eat your additional carbs after dinner, that is perfectly OK as well. Late in the day or after a workout is generally the best time to refuel your body with carbohydrates. Tracking your personal energy levels is the greatest approach to figure out when to eat more carbs in your meal plan.

Recommendation for Carbohydrate Consumption per Day

75–150 grammes of activity

100–200 grammes of highly active protein

100+ grammes if you're pregnant or nursing.

Estimates are based on the information available at the time. Adjust your carbohydrate intake if you find yourself unable to maintain your activity level.

Consider adding these carbohydrate sources if you are pregnant or nursing. Don't limit them in the hope of improving outcomes. It is not required to restrict these items any farther in order to achieve the program's goal of a healthy body and healthy baby. To boost your milk supply and stave off exhaustion, eat more carbohydrate-heavy foods like those listed here.

more information for those with autoimmune diseases

THIS CHANGE MAY BE PERFECT FOR YOU, IF

be diagnosed with an autoimmune illness or suspect you may have one.

For individuals who do not meet the above-mentioned modification criteria, you will be removing from your diet certain foods that are deemed Yes foods by the Autoimmune Modifications. As well as being common allergies, these foods tend to be digestion-inhibiting. Immune function can be boosted by better digestion. To test how your body reacts to these foods if you have an autoimmune problem, I strongly recommend eliminating them for the 21 days of this programme and then reintroducing them and tracking any changes.

EGGS

remove from your dietary intake

See this page for suggestions on how to substitute eggs in your cooking.

There are several types of nuts and seeds.

remove food and snacks from your diet

Included in this category are nuts in all forms (whole, nut butter, sesame, and seed butter). If a recipe can handle the substitution or omission of nuts, they are highlighted in the instructions.

Spices with Nightshade Vegetables

remove from your dietary intake

Spices like paprika (and cayenne pepper) and chilli powder are also included in this list of ingredients. It is stated if the recipe can handle the substitution or deletion of nightshades in the ingredients list.

Oatmeal and banana vanilla bean bread

Preparation time: 15 minutes; cooking time: 15 minutes; servings: 4 nuts; chilling time: 3 hours

EGGS

NIGHTSHADES

FODMAPS

SEAFOOD

2 hens' eggs

1 pod of vanilla extract

1 3/4 cups of coconut milk, either canned or handmade, 14.5 ounces (see here)

A quarter cup of water

1 sliced banana with a green tip

1 tsp. cinnamon powder 1 tsp. sea salt

Optional garnishes: sliced bananas or additional coconut milk, 1/4 cup chia seeds chopped almonds (if nut-free, eliminate).

You'll need to whisk the eggs in a small bowl and place the bowl near to the stove. Using a paring knife and the tip of one side of a vanilla bean pod, remove the seeds. In a medium saucepan, combine the scraped-out seeds, bean pod, coconut milk, and water. Heat slowly, stirring frequently. Stir more regularly as the mixture reaches a simmer and continue to simmer for another 5 minutes. Using a spoon, scrape out the vanilla bean pod and toss it out. While whisking rapidly, slowly pour a ladleful of the heated coconut milk mixture into the eggs. Continue to whisk as you add the coconut milk and egg combination back into the saucepan, making sure to scrape the bottom as needed. Stirring occasionally, cook for 5 to 10 minutes, or until a spoon dipped in the mixture comes out clean.

In a blender, combine the rest of the ingredients, then add the banana and blend for about a minute or two. Chia seeds and cinnamon are added and pulsed a few times or until they are uniformly distributed.

At least three hours, preferably overnight, refrigerate the mixture in four serving bowls, jars, or glasses. Coconut milk, chopped almonds, banana slices, or additional coconut milk can be added to the top of the smoothie. In order to serve the dish warm, reheat it in a pot over low heat.

TIP FOR INGREDIENTS

You may see a list of suggested manufacturers here.

EGG-FREE?

Don't bother with the egg. To make the smoothie, combine all ingredients in a blender and blend until smooth. Add the chia seeds last. Refrigerate for at least four hours before serving. The texture will be more like a thick, creamy yoghurt.

Chapter Four

skillet of carrots and apples

Breakfast hash made with a skillet of carrots and apples

15 minutes to prepare; 25 to 30 minutes to cook; 4 servings

NUTS

EGGS

NIGHTSHADES

FODMAPS

SEAFOOD

Chopped up four slices of bacon

a pound of peeled and sliced carrots (2 cups shredded)

An apple, peeled and cored (1 cup shredded)

The equivalent of one pound of ground chicken, turkey, or pork

1/4 cup Italian Sausage Spice Mixture (see here) salt & pepper to your liking

Cook the bacon for 8 to 10 minutes, tossing periodically, in a large skillet or sauté pan over medium heat, until the fat has rendered and the meat is crispy. The carrots and apple can be shredded in tandem with the bacon as it cooks.

Using a heat-safe spatula or wooden spoon, crumble up the chicken and add it to the pan once the bacon has finished cooking. Cook for about 8 minutes, stirring periodically, or until the meat is well cooked (there should be no pink remaining). If necessary, adjust the flavour with additional Spice Blend and/or salt & pepper.

Add the carrots and apple to the pan and lower the heat to medium-low. Cover and cook for about 5 minutes, or until the carrots are fork-tender. Before serving, remove the pan's lid and let any remaining liquid evaporate.

Replace the carrots with shredded sweet potatoes.

Chapter Five

green smoothie with apple and ginger

THE COOKING TIME IS 5 MINUTES; THE SERVING IS 2

NUTS

EGGS

NIGHTSHADES

FODMAPS

SEAFOOD

2-cups spinach in a bag

Almond milk or 2 cups of canned* or homemade full-fat coconut milk (here)

1 cup of ice

Lemon juice from half an avocado

Fresh ginger, peeled and minced, is all that is needed for this recipe.

Cut up a green apple into cubes.

14 to 12 cup of liquid

TIP FOR INGREDIENTS

You may see a list of suggested manufacturers here.

Blend everything together until smooth, adding more water if necessary. Blend for about a minute and a half.

Chapter Six

Smoothie of apple pie

TIME REQUIRED FOR PREP: 5 MINUTES

NUTS

EGGS

NIGHTSHADES

FODMAPS

SEAFOOD

Full-fat coconut milk, either canned or homemade, should be used in this recipe (see here)

A quarter cup of water

Cut up a green apple into cubes.

Almond butter, 2 tbsp.

Extract of vanilla flavouring : 1 teaspoon

1 1/2 tsp. cinnamon powder

2 tsp nutmeg, a few ice cubes for garnish (optional)

Whey protein powder made from 100 percent grass-fed whey and other single-ingredient powders** (optional)

TIPS FOR USING INGREDIENTS

A list of the best brands may be found at this link.

Review your Yes/No Foods List for more information on protein powder.

Non-Nut?

Coconut or Sunbutter can be used in place of almond butter.

A blender is all that is needed to get the job done.

Coconut butter is a better substitute for almond butter than almond butter.

Chapter Seven

smoothie with a hint of pumpkin spice

TIME REQUIRED FOR PREP: 5 MINUTES

NUTS

EGGS

NIGHTSHADES

FODMAPS

SEAFOOD

Full-fat coconut milk, either canned or homemade, should be used in this recipe (see here)

A quarter cup of water

1 frozen banana with a green tip

14 cup of pumpkin in a can

Extract of vanilla flavouring : 1 teaspoon

Cinnamon powder: 1 tbsp

Spices from a pumpkin pie a teeny-tiny piece of ice (optional)

Whey protein powder made from 100 percent grass-fed whey and other single-ingredient powders** (optional)

TIPS FOR USING INGREDIENTS

You may see a list of suggested manufacturers here.

Review your Yes/No Foods List for more information on protein powder.

A blender is all that is needed to get the job done.

Using sweet potatoes instead of pumpkin is an option.

Chapter Eight

breakfast in a southwestern style skillet

15 minutes to prepare; 25 minutes to cook; 4 servings

NUTS

EGGS

NIGHTSHADES

FODMAPS

SEAFOOD

Coconut oil or any other cooking fat*: 1 tbsp

1/2 cup red onion, chopped

Yellow bell peppers in half a cup

Red bell peppers in half a cup of chopped form

The minced jalapeo pepper (optional)

The equivalent of one pound of ground beef or bison, turkey, or fowl

Southwestern Spice Blend (see here), divided into 2 tbsp

Shredded parsnips of four large ones (4 cups)

Chopped green chiles in a 4-ounce can

6 eggs, to taste, with sea salt and pepper

2-3 Tbsp Avocado Crema (or something like that) (see here)

4 sprigs of fresh cilantro, chopped

Add the onion, bell peppers, and jalapenos to a large oven-safe pan and sauté for 1 minute over medium-high heat in the melted coconut oil. Add 1 tablespoon of the Spice Blend to the crumbled ground meat and mix until evenly distributed. The beef should be browned and almost cooked through after about 10 minutes of cooking.

Make sure to incorporate all of the remaining Spice Blend into the parsnips and the green chilies before serving. The parsnips should soften in approximately 3 to 5 minutes, but don't allow them to get too mushy.

Preheat the broiler to low and the oven rack to the top.

The meat-parsnip combination should be divided into six equal portions, each of which should be topped with an egg. The whites should be cooked completely and the yolks should be the desired doneness, so place the pan in the broiler for around 5 minutes.

Garnish with Avocado Crema and cilantro and season with salt & pepper to taste before serving.

TIP FOR INGREDIENTS

Use this link to see which cooking fats are best.

quiche that's worth the wait without a crust

10 minutes of prep time; 45 minutes of cooking time (plus 45 minutes for caramelised onions) for 4 servings;

EGGS

NIGHTSHADES

FODMAPS

SEAFOOD

Onions Caramelized (see here)

A baking dish should be greased with 1 tablespoon of cooking fat*.

8 pieces of chopped bacon

Salt and black pepper to taste on eight eggs

If you haven't previously, make the Caramelized Onions.

Set the temperature of the oven to 350 degrees Fahrenheit. A 9-by-11-inch casserole dish should be prepared.

Cook the bacon for 8 to 10 minutes, stirring occasionally, in a large skillet set over medium heat until the fat has rendered and the meat is crispy. The grease can be left in the pan while the bacon is drained using a slotted spoon and a paper towel.

Add salt and pepper to a bowl of beaten eggs and whisk until smooth. Add the Caramelized Onions and bacon to the beaten eggs and mix well. Bake for 30-40 minutes, or until the eggs swell up and the edges brown and pull away from the pan's sides, in the prepared casserole dish.

Once defrosted overnight, this quiche can be frozen and reheated in a toaster oven.

Salad greens or sautéed greens go well with this dish as well.

TIP FOR INGREDIENTS

The best cooking oils can be found here.

Chef's Notes

If you're looking for a quick way to create caramelised onions, this is it! For recipes like this and the BBQ Sauce here, I suggest making a double batch.

Chapter Nine

frittata with a pizza crust

TIME TO PREPARE 15 MINUTES, COOK 35 MINUTES, SERVE 6

NUTS

EGGS

NIGHTSHADES

FODMAPS

SEAFOOD

Meat that weighs 1 1/2 pounds

Italian Sausage Spice Blend: 1 tbsp (see here)

8 hens' eggs

salt, divided into 14 teaspoonfuls

Half a black peppercorn

Tomato sauce in a half cup measure

12 tsp. fresh basil

A quarter of a teaspoon of oregano

Garlic granules: 1/8 teaspoon

1 tbsp. fat for cooking*

1 thinly chopped bell pepper

5 sliced mushrooms

3-scallion (green onion) slices

Olives cut into half-cup portions

TIP FOR INGREDIENTS

The best cooking oils can be found here.

Prepare a 400°F oven.

Medium-high heat in an oven-safe skillet is needed to get the skillet up to temperature. Ground pork and spices should be mixed together in a bowl while the skillet heats up. In a mixing bowl, combine the ingredients and mix thoroughly until the spices are evenly dispersed. Break up the meat with a heat-safe spatula or wooden spoon as it cooks for about 10 minutes, until it's no longer pink in the centre. To save time, take the pork out of the pan and set it aside. (There is no need to clean the pan; you will reuse it.)

Salt and pepper the eggs in a small bowl and then add them to the mixture. Salt, basil, oregano, and granulated garlic are all mixed into the tomato sauce in a separate small bowl. Both bowls should be put away.

Add the bell pepper to the same pan you used to cook the pork and cook it until it begins to soften, about 5 minutes. Remove from the heat and set aside. Take out of the heat and stir in the mushrooms for 2 minutes, or until they begin to soften. Toss in the meat, green onions, and olives back into the pan and toss to incorporate them all.

To ensure that the eggs are evenly distributed throughout, tilt the pan back and forth while pouring. Gently whisk the ingredients together if necessary to ensure that they are evenly distributed. Allow to cook for about 5 minutes, or until the edges are beginning to firm up.

Then place the pan in the oven and bake for 8 to 10 minutes, or until the eggs are cooked through. Make a small cut in the middle of the frittata with a knife and see whether any raw egg comes out; if so, continue cooking for another 2 to 3 minutes.

Slice and serve after 5 minutes of resting.

If you don't want to use pork, you can substitute cooked spinach for it.

Chapter Ten

frittata with mushrooms and green onions

It takes 10 minutes to prep, 30 minutes to cook, and 4 people to eat.

NUTS

EGGS

NIGHTSHADES

FODMAPS

SEAFOOD

Mushrooms: 8 cremini

Bacon fat, ghee or coconut oil 1 tablespoon sea salt and black pepper

4 scallions (green onions) sliced thinly

Thyme dried, 12 tsp (optional)

8 hens' eggs

Coconut milk, canned or homemade, or Almond Milk, 2 tablespoons (here)

Serving Size of Sweetener-Free Ketchup (see here; optional, omit for nightshade free)

Set the temperature of the oven to 350 degrees Fahrenheit.

Slice the mushrooms into small strips and place them on a baking dish. Melt the cooking fat in a large cast-iron (or other oven-safe) skillet over medium heat. About 10 minutes into cooking the mushrooms, add a pinch of salt and pepper and continue to stir until they have shed their moisture and browned in the fat. Cook the green onions and dried thyme for one more minute after adding them to the pan with the olive oil.

Mix the eggs and milk together in a bowl, then season generously with salt and pepper. For 2 minutes, fry the eggs in the pan with the vegetables on medium heat. Then, transfer the skillet to the oven to finish cooking. Puff the eggs and brown the edges and pull away from the pan's sides for 15 to 20 minutes.

Serve with Sweetener-Free Ketchup, which you can find by clicking here.

Chapter Eleven

a biscuit and sausage breakfast sandwich

10 minutes to prepare; 15 to 18 minutes to cook; 4 servings

NUTS

EGGS

NIGHTSHADES

FODMAPS

SEAFOOD

SAUSAGE IS NEEDED FOR THIS

ground pork or other meat, about a pound

Add 2 teaspoons of the Spice Blend for Breakfast Sausage (see here)

As needed, 1 to 2 tablespoons of cooking fat.

Sliced sea salt and black pepper over 2 bell peppers

Eggs from four hens

Buns made with "Buttermilk" (see here)

Make sure you don't over-mix the meat and Spice Blend in a mixing bowl, otherwise the meat will turn tough. Make four patties out of the beef and cook them in a big skillet over medium heat for four minutes on each side, or until they're done. Removing the patties from the griddle and discarding the fat is optional. Add more fat if necessary (you should have about 1 tablespoon of fat in the pan).

Salt and pepper the bell peppers before adding them to the pan. Cook the peppers for about 5 minutes, or until they're tender and starting to colour.

Over medium-low heat, cook the eggs to your preference, adding cooking grease to the skillet if necessary to keep them from sticking, either in a separate skillet in the same one as the peppers. Depending on how you prepare the eggs, the cooking time can range from 3 to 5 minutes.)

Assemble your sandwich by putting one bun on the platter and then adding the peppers, sausage, and egg on top. Make additional burgers with the remaining ingredients.

It's NIGHTSHODE OUT!

Instead of using the Breakfast Sausage Spice Blend, try the Italian Sausage Spice Blend (see here) and eliminate the bell peppers altogether.

Chef's Notes

Cook the sausage, peppers, and buns ahead of time and cook the eggs to order in the morning while reheating the other ingredients in a 300°F oven for 10 minutes to make this recipe quick and easy for your morning breakfast.

pancakes made with butternut squash

SERVES 4 AND RETURNS 16 4-INCH PANCAKE NUTS FOR PREP AND COOKING OVER A 15-MINUTE PERIOD WITH AN ADDITIONAL 20-MINUTE COOKING TIME FOR THE SQUASH

EGGS

NIGHTSHADES

FODMAPS

SEAFOOD

1 cup mashed butternut squash, prepared by steaming and mashing it

Eggs from four hens

There are 2 quarts of almond flour

Full-fat coconut milk, either canned or homemade, should be used in this recipe (see here)

4 tbsp. ground cinnamon per serving

One-half teaspoon nutmeg powder

2 cloves, crushed, to taste

Ground ginger is around half a teaspoon.

Cocoa powder*: 2 teaspoons

Using 4 tbsp of pure vanilla extract,

1 tbsp. of coconut oil per serving

With a spoonful of the Spiced Buttery Apple Spread (see here)

Blend all items except coconut oil and Spiced Buttery Apple Spread until smooth in a food processor or big blender.

Mix all of the ingredients together in a large bowl and form a dough by hand. In 4-inch circles, drop approximately a fourth of a cup of batter at a time (the batter should yield about 16 pancakes total). Depending on your pan, this could take anywhere from 1 1/2 to 2 minutes. To make pancakes easier to flip, most of the cooking is done on this side. Flip each pancake with a spatula slipped under it in a flash. Cook for an additional minute, or until the meat is no longer pink in the middle.

Spiced Buttery Apple Spread is a great accompaniment.

TIP FOR INGREDIENTS

You may see a list of suggested manufacturers here.

Chef's Notes

To get the pancakes to the right size, you'll need a spoon to distribute the batter in the pan after you drop it in.

Instead of butternut squash, try mashed sweet potatoes or plantains.

Chapter Twelve

grilled chicken

Cooking time is 30 to 35 minutes; serving size is 4 to 6 people.

NUTS

EGGS

NIGHTSHADES

FODMAPS

SEAFOOD

1 sliced yellow onion

Two sliced shallots

2 chopped or grated garlic cloves

4 limes' worth of juice

Extra-virgin olive oil in a tablespoon

Chili powder, 1 tsp.

a quarter teaspoon of salt from the sea

Half a black peppercorn

Boneless, skinless chicken thighs weighing 1 1/2 to 2 pounds

Basic Cauli-Rice with Cilantro (below), to serve

For garnish, use a lime wedged in half.

For garnish: 1/4 cup chopped fresh cilantro.

Toss the ingredients together in a big bowl, except for the chicken, Cauli-Rice, and garnishes. For at least an hour, marinate the chicken in a shallow, nonreactive container.

Pre-heat the oven to 375°F

Bake for 30 to 35 minutes, or until the chicken is white all the way through and reaches an internal temperature of 165°F.

Slice the chicken with two forks. Serve with Cilantro Cauli-Rice as a side dish. Fresh cilantro and lime wedges are perfect for garnishing this dish.

It's NIGHTSHODE OUT!

Chili powder is not necessary.

Chili powder is not necessary.

Chapter Thirteen

basic cauli-rice with cilantro

COOK TIME: 5 MINS • SERVING SIZE: 4 TO 6 MINUTES

NUTS

EGGS

NIGHTSHADES

FODMAPS

SEAFOOD

Cauliflower heads

1 tbsp. bacon fat or coconut oil.

salt & pepper to your liking

1/4 cup fresh cilantro, chopped finely

COLOR & VARIETY OPTIONAL ADD-ONS

as shown

Red onion chopped into 1/4 cup

quarter-cup yellow bell pepper, finely chopped (omit for nightshade free)

1 tbsp. bacon fat or coconut oil.

Cauliflower should be cut into large bits once the outer leaves and stem have been removed. Shred the cauliflower in the food processor or using a box grater.

In a small skillet, sauté the onion and pepper in 1 tablespoon of coconut oil or bacon grease for about 5 minutes or until they are tender and have golden brown edges.

Place the shredded cauliflower in a large skillet with the coconut oil or bacon fat and heat to a simmer over medium heat. Taste and adjust the seasonings. Cauliflower should be cooked through in about 5 minutes, stirring carefully to ensure that it doesn't burn.

Toss the chopped cilantro into the cauliflower before serving, and add the other add-ins if desired.

Leave off the bell peppers if you're making this.

Chapter Fourteen

pot pie with chicken

COOK TIME: 50 MINUTES • PREP TIME: 30 MINS • SERVINGS 4:

NUTS

EGGS

NIGHTSHADES

FODMAPS

SEAFOOD

CRUST

1 1/3 cups of almond flour

A half-cup of coconut flour.*

1/2 tsp. salt from the sea

whisked 2 eggs

Fractionated coconut oil or 10 tablespoons of butter or lard

FILLING

8 tbsp. ghee or butter

chopped 2 carrots, medium in size (1 cup)

1 medium diced onion (1 cup)

1 cup finely diced fresh green beans

Diced celery from two stalks (1 cup)

1 1/2 cups sliced cremini mushroom tops

More sea salt can be added if necessary.

Add more as necessary, but keep it to a minimum.

flour made from arrowroot

1 3/4 cups of canned or homemade full-fat coconut milk (approximately 14.5 ounces) (see here)

3 cups of Bone Broth, chicken (see here), and a little salt and pepper to taste

Dried parsley: 1 tbsp

1 tsp. thyme dried

chicken cooked and shredded to 3 cups (see Chef Note)

a single egg's white

2 tbsp. of liquid

Prepare a 400°F oven.

In a food processor, add the almond flour, coconut flour, and salt; pulse 4 to 5 times, or until well incorporated. This will be your crust. Blend in the eggs for 15 to 20 seconds, or until completely smooth. Shred the butter using a cheese grater from the freezer. Process 10 seconds with half of the grated butter in the processor. Just a few pulses are all that is needed to incorporate the second half of the butter (small pieces of butter will still be visible). Divide the mixture into four equal portions once it has been processed in the food processor. Wrap each piece individually in plastic wrap and refrigerate. Refrigerate the dough balls until they are firm.

Melt the butter in a pot over medium heat. Add the flour and cook for a few minutes. Onion and carrots should be cooked for 5 minutes, or until they are transparent. Then, add the green beans. Cook the celery and mushrooms for 3 to 5 minutes, or until the mushrooms are tender.

The salt, pepper, and arrowroot flour can be mixed together in a small bowl and then sprinkled over the vegetables. Stir the arrowroot flour into the mixture for about 2 minutes to ensure that it is thoroughly incorporated. Cook for 10 minutes, stirring occasionally, until the coconut milk and Bone Broth have thickened to a gravy-like consistency. Cook for an additional 5 to 10 minutes with the parsley, thyme, and shredded chicken, then remove from the heat and serve. Salt and pepper to taste, if necessary.

The pies are ready to be baked: Fill four 12-ounce ovenproof soufflé dishes or similar individual-sized dishes to the brim with the filling.

Discard any ice that may have formed on the pie dough and let it come to room temperature before rolling it out between two sheets of parchment paper to a thickness of approximately 1/4 inch. Roll out a piece of dough and gently set it on top of each baking dish. If there are any cracks, they should be forcefully pressed back together.

In a small bowl, combine the egg white and water. Apply the egg white mixture to the entire crust with a brush. Discard any uncooked crusts that have stuck to the pan after baking.

Bake the pot pies for 15 to 20 minutes, or until the tops are golden brown, on a rimmed sheet pan. Allow 10 to 15 minutes for the dish to cool completely before serving.

TIP FOR INGREDIENTS

You may see a list of suggested manufacturers here.

Chef's Notes

Alternatively, if you don't have any leftover chicken, simply bake 1 pound of bone-in, skinless chicken in a 350°F oven for 30-40 minutes until an internal temperature of 165°F is reached. Clean-ingredient store-bought rotisserie chicken can also be used.

Cooked crab flesh can be used in place of the chicken.

chicken adobo in the crock pot

Preparation time: 25 minutes; cooking time: 4 to 6 hours; servings: 4 nuts.

EGGS

NIGHTSHADES

FODMAPS

SEAFOOD

1-inch-thick slices of yellow onion

Peeled and finely sliced, a 2-inch piece of fresh ginger

1 peeled and finely sliced head of garlic (approximately 12 cloves)

Two bay leaves

1 3/4 cups of canned or homemade full-fat coconut milk (approximately 14.5 ounces) (see here)

A half-cup serving of coconut aminos

The vinegar is 1/3 cup of apple cider

For the chicken, add an additional 2 tablespoons of black pepper.

2 tbsp. fat for cooking**

bones-in thigh meat for 3 pounds

sodium chloride, or salt of the earth

Cauli-Rice with Garlic and Green Onions, for serving (see here)

Set your slow cooker on the lowest setting and add the onion, ginger, garlic and bay leaves. The coconut milk, coconut aminos, apple cider vinegar, and pepper should be mixed together in a bowl before being served.

In a skillet, heat the cooking fat to a high temperature. Place the skin-side-down chicken thighs in the skillet and liberally season the skin with salt and pepper. About 5 minutes of cooking time is required to get the skin golden brown.

Pour the coconut milk mixture over the chicken thighs and simmer on low for 8 to 10 hours.

Cook for four hours on high or six hours on low.

Take out the cooked chicken from the slow cooker, then bring the remaining sauce to a boil in a saucepan over medium-high heat and cook for 20 to 25 minutes to thicken or until the required thickness is attained, depending on your preference.

Garlic and Green Onion Cauli-Rice is a good accompaniment.

TIP FOR INGREDIENTS

You may see a list of suggested manufacturers here.

COOKING ADVICE

**(click here) for cooking fat recommendations.

Chapter Fifteen

The chicken in a lemon ginger sauce

COOKING TIME: 20 to 25 minutes; SERVINGS: 4

NUTS

EGGS

NIGHTSHADES

FODMAPS

SEAFOOD

A quarter-cup of coconut aminos

Ground ginger is around half a teaspoon.

a quarter teaspoon of salt from the sea

Black pepper in a quarter teaspoon

1 half-lemon, halved

Flour made from the arrowroot plant

Thighs, boneless and skinless, weighing 2 pounds

2 tbsp. ghee or coconut oil

8 thinly sliced scallions (1 cup)

As a finishing touch, sprinkle some sesame seeds on top.

The last touch is a teaspoon of cold-pressed sesame oil.

In order to serve, Asian Sautéed Greens (see here)

Set the temperature of the oven to 350 degrees Fahrenheit.

Combine all of the ingredients for the chicken marinade in a big mixing bowl: the coconut aminos, ginger, salt & pepper, half of the lemon's juice, and arrowroot flour. Let the chicken marinate for 5 minutes in the marinade.

In a large oven-safe skillet, melt the coconut oil over medium heat. Slice the remaining half of the lemon while the pan is heating up. It's time to put in the chicken and fry it for 2 minutes on each side when the oil is heated. Top with green onions, sesame seeds, and lemon slices before serving. A temperature of 165 degrees Fahrenheit is required for the chicken to be cooked through (no pink remains) and for the juices to run clear.

Sesame oil and sesame seeds can be added as a finishing touch.

Asian Sautéed Greens are a perfect complement to this dish.

TIP FOR INGREDIENTS

You may see a list of suggested manufacturers here.

The oil and seeds of sesame are not required in this recipe.

Chapter Sixteen

tandoori chicken skewers

PREP TIME 20 MINS (+ 3 OR MORE HRS TO MARINATE) • COOK TIME 20 MINS • SERVINGS 6 TO 8

NUTS

EGGS

NIGHTSHADES

FODMAPS

SEAFOOD

Canned or homemade full-fat coconut milk can be used in this recipe (see here)

Chop 12 a small red onion

Garlic cloves of three

1/4 cup freshly grated ginger

As much tomato paste as you like.

Ground coriander: 2 tbsp.

1 tbsp. cumin ground

One teaspoon of paprika.

1/2 tsp. salt from the sea

Four 1 1/2-inch cubed boneless, skinless chicken breasts (total weight: 2 pounds)

charcoal-grill skewers (see Kitchen Tip)

Using a blender or food processor, combine or process the ingredients, but do not add the chicken, until the marinade is smooth and creamy. Pour the coconut milk mixture over the chicken in a large zip-top bag or container. Refrigerate for at least three hours, if not all night, to provide the best flavour.

Pre-heat a grill or grill pan to high heat when you're ready to cook the chicken. Meanwhile, skewer 5-6 cubes of chicken per person while the grill is heating up. Place the skewers on the grill and lower the heat to medium. Each skewer should be grilled for 8 to 10 minutes before being flipped over; the chicken should come readily off the grates when the skewer is ready to be flipped. A last 10 to 12 minutes on the grill will ensure that the chicken is cooked thoroughly and reaches an internal temperature of 165°F.

Mini Sweet Potato Flatbreads (for Energy Modifications) and Moroccan Cauli-Rice Pilaf are excellent accompaniments to these skewers. (see here).

TIP FOR INGREDIENTS

You may see a list of suggested manufacturers here.

TIPS FOR THE KITCHEN

Keep wooden skewers off of the grill by soaking them in water for at least 15 minutes.

To prepare this dish, marinate swordfish for 15 to 20 minutes, or use a fish of a similar texture.

Chapter Seventeen

Zucchini noodles with chicken in a creamy tomato sauce

Preparation time: 15 minutes (including marinara and chicken preparation) • Cooking time: 15 minutes • Servings: 4

NUTS

EGGS

NIGHTSHADES

FODMAPS

SEAFOOD

a combination of 4 large or 8 little zucchinis, yellow squashes, or a single zucchini

There is only one recipe for this: Simple Marinara (see here)

1/4 cup canned* or homemade full-fat coconut milk (see here)

a pound of cooked boneless, skinless chicken breasts (see Chef Note)

Over medium-high heat, bring 1 inch of water to a boil in an enormous pot. In the pot, place a steamer basket to cook your vegetables.

You may use a portable julienne peeler or simply a standard vegetable peeler to shred the zucchini or yellow squash into noodles as the water comes to a boil (if using a regular peeler, the noodles will be wide and flat instead of spaghetti-shaped). 4 cups of noodles should enough. Steam the noodles for 3 minutes in a basket, then drain them in a colander to remove any remaining water as they cool down.

Warm the Simple Marinara and coconut milk in a large skillet over low heat. If you're using leftover chicken, simply reheat it.

Toss the zoodles with the sauce once it has heated through. Serve the zoodles and sauce with the chicken sliced into thin strips on top of the zoodles. If you like, you can slice up some smaller pieces and include them into the recipe.

TIP FOR INGREDIENTS

A list of the best brands may be found at this link.

Chef's Notes

Simply season boneless skinless chicken breasts with sea salt and black pepper and bake them in a 350°F oven until done, or use the breast meat from a clean-ingredient rotisserie chicken to make this dish if you don't have any on hand.

Cooked shrimp can be substituted for the chicken in this recipe.

Chapter Eighteen

Strips of chicken

15 minutes to prepare, 35-40 minutes to cook, 4 to 6 servings

NUTS

EGGS

NIGHTSHADES

FODMAPS

SEAFOOD

The flour is 1 cup of arrowroot

Almond flour, one-half cup

Salt and black pepper to taste

4 tbsp. minced garlic

1 and a half tsp. salt

paprika

Full-fat coconut milk, either canned or homemade, should be used (see here)

The hot sauce is 2 teaspoons

Cut four boneless, skinless chicken breasts into 1-inch strips (approximately 1 1/2 to 2 pounds total).

Melted half a cup of coconut oil

No-Honey Mustard Sauce, BBQ Sauce, or Sweetener-Free Ketchup can all be used to accompany a meal.

Prepare a 400°F oven. Use parchment paper to line a rimmed baking sheet.

Mix together the arrowroot flour, almond flour, pepper, granulated garlic, salt, and paprika in a broad, shallow bowl or dish. The hot sauce and coconut milk should be mixed together in a separate wide, shallow basin.

Use a paper towel to pat each piece of chicken down to remove any excess moisture. Each strip should be dipped in the coconut milk mixture and shaken to remove the excess. Coat the strip thoroughly with the dry mixture. Bake the coated chicken strips for 20 minutes on the prepared baking sheet. Melted coconut oil should be applied to the tops of each strip with a pastry or sauce brush. To ensure that the chicken is cooked through and no longer pink in the middle, bake for an additional 15 to 20 minutes.

You can serve it with BBQ Sauce, Sweetener Free Ketchup, or No-Honey Mustard Sauce.

TIP FOR INGREDIENTS

You may see a list of suggested manufacturers here.

Chapter Nineteen

chicken curry with apples in a salad

PER SERVING: 4 to 6 MINUTES

NUTS

EGGS

NIGHTSHADES

FODMAPS

SEAFOOD

Homemade Mayonnaise in a cup: (see here)

*Apple cider vinegar has a sour taste.

Curry powder in the colour of turmeric

4 cooked, cooled, and diced boneless, skinless chicken breasts (approximately 2 pounds total)

Diced red onion from a medium-sized red onion

3-scallion (green onion) slices

Sliced three celery stalks

Two sliced green apples

FOR YOUR USE

Mixed greens and/or mixed fruits and vegetables, such as jicama or cucumber slices

In a small bowl, combine the mayonnaise and apple cider vinegar. Whisk in the curry powder after adding it to the mayonnaise mixture. Combine the chicken with the red and green onions, celery, and apples in a large bowl. To make sure the chicken is completely covered, combine the mayonnaise and remaining ingredients in a large bowl and toss until well combined.

It's up to you what you'd like to accompany it with.

TIP FOR INGREDIENTS

You may see a list of suggested manufacturers here.

Instead of chicken, use canned tuna or salmon.

barbecue chicken: 5 minutes to prepare; 25 to 30 minutes to cook; 4 servings

NUTS

EGGS

NIGHTSHADES

FODMAPS

SEAFOOD

A total of 4 chicken thigh halves with skin on or 8 chicken thighs

salt and pepper from the sea

2-cups of BBQ Sauce (optional) (see here)

Grill or grill pans should be preheated to high heat. Pat the chicken dry after rinsing.

Turn the heat down to medium-low. Place the skin-side down of the chicken on the grill and season generously with salt and pepper. Baste with the BBQ Sauce after 10 minutes of cooking, then flip over and continue cooking for an additional 10 minutes. If necessary, continue cooking for another 15 to 20 minutes or until the internal temperature reaches 165°F. Make sure the chicken is cooked through and the sauce isn't scorching by placing it in an oven at 350 degrees Fahrenheit or on a grill pan and cooking it until done.

Add extra BBQ Sauce to the plate for dipping if desired.

Chapter Twenty

Cottage pie with meat and bacon

TIME TO PREPARE 15 MINUTES, COOK FOR 50 MINUTES, SERVE 6

NUTS

EGGS

NIGHTSHADES

FODMAPS

SEAFOOD

2 1/2 pounds of medium-sized butternut squash

Coconut oil or ghee is a good substitute.

salt and pepper from the sea

bacon, cut into 1/2-inch pieces, 8 slices plus extra for adornment, if you like chopped 2 carrots, medium in size (1 cup)

1 cup of green beans, chopped up

Diced half of a medium yellow onion (1 cup)

2 pounds of bison or beef mashed up

Blended Smoky Spice, 4 tbsp (see here)

Pre-heat the oven to 375°F

Cut the butternut squash in half lengthwise after peeling it with a vegetable peeler. Remove the seeds and chop the 1-inch pieces into smaller pieces. Prepare a steamer basket and a saucepan of water with 1 to 2 inches of depth. Fork-tender squash takes 15 to 20 minutes to steam on high heat. Grind the squash in a food processor till smooth, seasoning to taste, while it is still warm.

In a large skillet over medium heat, fry the bacon until the fat has drained off, about 8 to 10 minutes. With a slotted spoon, remove the bacon from the skillet and set it aside, with the bacon fat remaining in the pan. In a skillet, sauté the carrots and green beans over medium heat for 5 minutes, stirring occasionally. Continue to cook until the carrots are just starting to soften, about 5 more minutes after adding the onion. Use a spatula to break up any clumps of meat and to mix the meat and Spice Blend together in the pan before cooking. Cook the beef and carrots until they are tender but not mushy.

Use a deep pie plate or a 9-by-13-inch rectangle baking dish to place the meat mixture in the oven to bake for an hour or two. The butternut squash puree should be placed on top of the bacon, with the exception of a few pieces for decoration. After 20 minutes, check the top for browning. Add a little extra bacon to the top.

Instead of butternut squash, use cooked and mashed sweet potatoes as a topping.

Chapter Twenty-one

pork smothered in cinnamon and fennel

15-minute prep time; 8+-hour cook time; 8 servings

NUTS

EGGS

NIGHTSHADES

FODMAPS

SEAFOOD

Peeled and roughly sliced two green apples

coarsely chopped 1 bulb of fennel (save fronds for garnish)

1 finely sliced small yellow onion

Garlic cloves, roughly minced, 4

2 tbsp. of cinnamon powder

1 tsp. salt from the sea

Peppercorns: 1 tbsp

1/8 teaspoon cumin seed powder

a tablespoon of gluten-free brown mustard*

Apple cider vinegar, divided into four equal servings

Bacon fat or coconut oil, about two tablespoons

Pork shoulder or butt (3 lb.) roast

A quarter cup of water

2 sticks of cinnamon

In the bottom of a slow cooker, combine the apples, fennel, onion, and garlic. Mix together the ground cinnamon, salt, pepper, cumin, mustard, and 1 tablespoon of apple cider vinegar in a small mixing dish to produce a paste. Spread the spice paste over the top and edges of the pork after spreading the bacon fat over it. Make sure the pork is placed in the slow cooker on top of the vegetables. In a slow cooker, place the cinnamon sticks and the remaining 3 tablespoons of apple cider vinegar.

If the beef isn't falling apart readily with a fork, cook it for another 8 hours on low heat. If desired, top with the fennel fronds you set aside earlier.

TIP FOR INGREDIENTS

A list of the best brands may be found at this link.

TIPS FOR THE KITCHEN

A slow cooker? It's all good! In an enamelled cast-iron Dutch oven set to 200°F for 8 hours, or until the meat flakes readily with a fork, prepare this dish.

beef flank steak marinated in asian ginger sauce

It takes 10 minutes to prepare and 18 minutes to cook, with 4 to 6 nuts per serving.

EGGS

NIGHTSHADES

FODMAPS

SEAFOOD

1 Tbsp Garlic Chili Sauce (see here)

A single lemon's peel, or (1 tablespoon)

Fresh ginger, chopped or grated, 1 (2-inch) piece (2 tablespoons)

Garlic minced or grated in 2 teaspoons

A half-cup serving of coconut aminos

a quarter teaspoon of salt from the sea

Flank steak, 1 to 1 1/2 pounds

1/4 cup sesame seed oil, cold-pressed

Serving a spicy slaw (see here)

The only things left are the flank steak, a drizzle of sesame oil, and the cole slaw. Assemble the marinade ingredients and pour them over the flank beef in a zip-top plastic bag. Make sure the meat is well-coated. Seal the bag by removing all of the air. Refrigerate for at least three hours before preparing.

Grill or grill pans should be preheated to high heat. Removing the steak from the marinade bag and discarding the remaining marinade is necessary. The steak should be cooked for 8 minutes before being flipped. In order to achieve the appropriate amount of doneness, cook for an additional 8 to 10 minutes. Ten minutes after removing from the heat, cover the dish and allow it to rest before serving.

Serve the sesame oil-drizzled steak with Spicy Slaw.

TIP FOR INGREDIENTS

You may see a list of suggested manufacturers here.

Chapter Twenty-two

Larb of meat

(thai lettuce wraps)

20-minute prep time; 10- to 12-minute cook time; and number of servings

NUTS

EGGS

NIGHTSHADES

FODMAPS

SEAFOOD

DUE TO THE FILLING

A squeeze of one lime

Amount of 2 Tbsp Coconut Amino Acid*

a teaspoon of fish sauce

1. one lemongrass strand

The cooking fat in a tablespoon**

2 minced shallots (2/3 cup)

The minced garlic of two cloves

2 thinly sliced Thai red chilies (or other hot red chilies) or other hot red chilies, as desired

Two limes' worth of zest

Meat or shrimp that weighs 1 1/2 pounds

TO USE AS SAUCE

juice of two limes

The fish sauce is 2 teaspoons

1 Tbsp Garlic Chili Sauce (see here)

Individual leaves of butter lettuce from a single huge head

Optional FINISHES

2 tablespoons finely chopped fresh cilantro and/or mint

Squeeze the juice of 1 lime over the wraps before serving.

Pour the lime juice, coconut aminos, and fish sauce into a small bowl and mix well. Dispose of. Leave a 4-inch piece of lemongrass after removing the base (the white end) and the upper third or half of the green part. After that, mince the lemongrass after removing any tough or dry outer layers. Melt the frying grease in a large skillet over medium heat. One minute later, add the shallots and garlic. Stir in the chilies, lemongrass, and lime zest and heat for 30 seconds, or until they begin to release their fragrance. After crumbling the meat into the skillet, heat for 5 to 8 minutes, stirring frequently to prevent sticking and to brown the meat evenly. Cook the meat for an extra minute after adding the lime juice mixture and stirring it in.

In a small bowl, combine the lime juice, fish sauce, and Garlic Chili Paste and whisk until smooth.

Garnish with mint or cilantro and lime wedges, if desired, and serve in a butter lettuce leaf.

TIP FOR INGREDIENTS

A list of the best brands may be found at this link.

Chef's Notes

**(click here) for cooking fat recommendations.

SEAFOOD-FREE?

The fish sauce should be omitted from the recipe entirely.

Instead of beef, use chopped/ground shrimp.

Chapter Twenty-three

Root vegetables and mushrooms are added to the pot roast

15 minutes of prep time, 8+ hours of cooking time, and 4 servings per recipe

NUTS

EGGS

NIGHTSHADES

FODMAPS

SEAFOOD

1 tbsp. fat for cooking*

Onion powder is half a teaspoon.

Garlic granules: 1/8 teaspoon

1 tsp. salt from the sea

Peppercorns: 1 tbsp

Bottom round roast weighing 1 1/2 pounds

1 and a half cups beef bone broth with garlic cloves (see here)

Onion slices of a medium size

Carrots of an extra-large size, chopped (3 to 4 cups)

1 large parsnip, chopped (1 1/2 cups)

Quartered mushrooms from six to eight mushrooms

1 tbsp. vinegar, such as apple cider or balsamic

More fresh rosemary can be added to the dish as needed.

This recipe calls for half a teaspoon of dried thyme.

OPTIONAL ADDITIONS.

Crushed or chopped tomatoes, or Sweetener-Free Ketchup (see here) (omit for nightshade-free)

a peeled and cut green apple

Melt the cooking fat in a cast-iron or stainless-steel skillet over high heat. Stir together onion powder and garlic granules with salt and pepper in a small basin while the pan heats, then liberally season the beef all over with this spice combination. Cook the meat for 2 minutes on each side in a skillet over high heat. In a crock pot, combine the seared beef with the Bone Broth and other ingredients such as onion and carrots and parsnips and mushrooms and vinegar. If using, combine with the ketchup, chopped or crushed tomatoes, and/or apple.

Stirring occasionally, simmer for at least eight hours or until the meat is easily torn apart with a fork

As soon as you've cooked your meat and drained any excess liquid from it, use a blender to puree 1/2 cup of cooked carrots and parsnips in high speed for 1 to 2 minutes until smooth.

CHESS MENTIONS

*Recommended fats for cooking can be found here.

skewers of satay meat

Cooking time ranges from 10 to 15 minutes, depending on how long it takes to marinate. • There are 4 servings in total.

NUTS

EGGS

NIGHTSHADES

FODMAPS

SEAFOOD

In order to marinate

Sliced lemongrass from a huge stem (2 tablespoons)

A quarter of a cup of chopped shallots

The minced garlic of two cloves

a dash of hot sauce

Ginger chopped into a quarter to half a teaspoon

1 tsp. turmeric powder

Coriander, ground to taste, 1 teaspoon

1 tbsp. cumin ground

Coconut aminos*: 3 teaspoons of the stuff

Somewhere between three and six tablespoons of the stuff

1 smashed cardamom pod

1/4 cup canned* or homemade full-fat coconut milk (see here)

salt and pepper from the sea

One-and-a-half pounds

TO USE AS SAUCE

3 tbsp. almond butter

1/4 cup coconut aminos*

1 tablespoon of canned or homemade full-fat coconut milk (see here)

Fish sauce*: 5 to 6 drops*

Onion powder is half a teaspoon.

Skewers, approximately 12–18

For garnish: 1/4 cup chopped fresh cilantro.

For garnish, use a lime wedged in half.

Set out a shallow bowl of water and put 12 to 18 wooden skewers within.

Prepare the marinade: In a large bowl, combine all of the marinade's components.

Slice the meat into 1/2-inch slices against the grain. Toss the steak in the marinade in a large bowl until well coated. Marinate for thirty minutes.

To make the sauce, combine all of the ingredients in a small mixing dish and whisk until smooth.

Take the time to heat up your grill or grill pan. Place each steak strip on a skewer and cook it on the grill until it's done. The skewers should be cooked in batches for around 2 to 3 minutes on each side, turning once. For every skewer, repeat this process. Serve with the sauce garnished with cilantro and lime slices.

CPSIA information can be obtained
at www.ICGtesting.com
Printed in the USA
LVHW060214160722
723616LV00015B/774

9 781804 768860